LOW CARB

Don't starve! How to fit into your old jeans in 7 days without starving with a Low Carb & High Protein Diet

Table of Contents

Introduction

Thank you very much for downloading this book, *"Low Carb – Don't starve! How to fit into your old jeans in 7 days without starving with a Low Carb & High Protein Diet"*. I congratulate you for taking this step so that you can become more enlightened. This book has actionable strategies on how to lose weight by simply adopting a low carb, high protein diet.

Carbohydrates, as other nutrients, serve a purpose. No matter what activity your body performs, energy is needed. Carbohydrates aid in regulating the circulation of sugar so that energy reaches every cell. Among other things, carbohydrates enable your body to absorb calcium and provide nutrients for the digestion of food. Additionally, your brain cells need energy from carbohydrates to function properly.

We are aware of the importance of carbohydrates and I am not disputing their significance. What I am disputing, is taking a diet that is rich in carbs especially refined carbohydrates.

Currently, our diet is so high in carbohydrates that it is no wonder we are dealing with a wide array of lifestyle diseases like diabetes, high blood pressure and heart disease among others. While carbohydrates are great since they are the main source of fuel for your body, the excess consumption of carbohydrates that we are notorious for, is not good for you. Therefore, if you want to reset your body and lose a few pounds while you are at it, a low carb diet is good for you.

If you want to learn more about a low-carb diet, this book will provide all the information you need and much more.

You will learn what a low-carb diet is, how many daily carbohydrate grams you need to take in a day, what you need to eat more and what intake to reduce, as well as some tasty recipes to get you started. I hope you enjoy this book and thank you for downloading.

Why A Low Carb High Protein Diet

A low carb diet simply restricts carbohydrates to less than 20-45% of your total daily caloric intake. Therefore, if you need to take 1200 calories, then only 240-540 calories should come from carbohydrates. This means you will reduce your intake of carbohydrates like grains, starchy vegetables, and fruits and eat more foods high in fat and protein like poultry, meat, eggs, fish, non-starchy vegetables, seeds, nuts, cheese, and vegetables low in carbohydrates such as chard, spinach, kale and collards.

I am sure you are probably wondering why the low carb diet when there are many different kinds of diet to help you lose weight. This makes it important to understand how the low carb diet works. Normally, once you take a meal high in carbohydrates, the carbohydrates are broken down into glucose, which is the principal energy. Therefore, as long as there is a ready supply of glucose, your body will not tap into your reserves. The essence behind a low carb diet is that when you limit the amount of carbohydrates you take, you force your body to burn muscle and fats for energy. In order to avoid your body breaking down muscles for energy, it is advisable for you take a high protein diet to provide the body with the amount of protein it requires then it will turn to fats for energy. In addition, after taking a meal high in carbohydrates, insulin is usually produced, as it is the hormone that helps the body cells to utilize glucose. It is also a fat storing hormone. This means that high levels of glucose trigger high levels of insulin to be released, which then leads to more glucose being stored as fat. This means reducing the amount of carbohydrates you take in a meal can greatly reduce the amount of insulin, thus reducing the total amount of extra fat stored. Other benefits of a low carb diet include improved energy levels owing to no sugar crashes, better mood, improved stress management, prevention of diabetes, obesity, blood pressure, and heart diseases.

The body cells meticulously allot the amount of carbs that is required. What is not needed, shows up on your hips, waist or thighs. Therefore, you should be as meticulous and detailed, about what you partake, rather than allowing your body cells to show you what will happen with the excess amount. It is important to monitor your carbs intake by recording what you have eaten. My aim is not only to ensure that you fit into your old pair of jeans but to empower you to implement healthier habits. You have to be disciplined and abide to your prescribed meals.

So, how many grams of carbohydrates should you be taking on a low carb diet? A low carb diet limits carbohydrates intake to between 50 -150 grams per day. For example, if you effortlessly want to lose weight while allowing for a bit of carbs in the diet, you are required to take 50-100 grams of carbohydrates per day. However, if you need to quickly lose weight, it is advisable to take about 20-50 grams of carbohydrates in a day though this may not be recommended as a long-term strategy. In most cases, after taking 20-50 grams daily, most people increase their carbohydrate intake.

What To Eat

Meat: Chicken, pork, lamb, beef and many others

Fish: Trout, salmon, haddock and many others

Eggs: Omega-3 enriched or pastured eggs are best

Avocado

Vegetables: Spinach, cauliflower, broccoli, carrots and many non-starchy vegetables

Fruits: Oranges, apples, pears, blueberries, strawberries

Nuts and seeds: Almonds, walnuts, sunflower seeds

Fats and healthy oils: Coconut oil, butter, lard, olive oil and cod fish liver oil, olive oil

Milk

Legumes: Beans, lentils, peas

High-Fat Dairy: Cheese, butter, heavy cream, yogurt

Note: If you need to lose weight, be careful with the cheese and nuts because you can easily overeat them. Do not eat more than one piece of fruit per day.

There are different types of fat: the good and the bad. Using the bad type of fat, increases the harmful type of cholesterol, creates inflammation and it is associated with health problems.

The healthy type of fat helps your body with digestion, the optimal functioning of the brain and the absorption of minerals and vitamins. This type of fat is found in nuts and avocados and the fat sources listed.

It is important to include Omega-3 fatty acids in your diet. They are vital fats because the body cannot produce them. They are essential as they create hormones that curb blood clotting and play an integral role in your body cells' performance.

Sources of Omega-3 are healthy oils; fish such as salmon, mackerel, and sardines; nuts such as walnuts and sunflower seeds; and dark leafy vegetables such as spinach, kale and broccoli. Omega-3 stabilizes the rhythm of your heart and lowers your blood pressure.

Protein is very important to your diet as it facilitates a strong immune system, maintains the balance of fluid and is used as a source of energy by your body. Muscle growth and structure and the nervous system are dependent on protein. Protein is found in soy products, dairy products, legumes, meat and fish.

What Not To Eat Or Reduce Intake

Sugar

Grains: Breads, Wheat, barley, spelt, rye and pastas.

Trans Fats: Hydrogenated or partially hydrogenated oils

Vegetable Oils: Cottonseed, soybean, sunflower, grape seed, corn, safflower and canola oils

Artificial Sweeteners: Cyclamates, Aspartame, Saccharin, Acesulfame Potassium, and Sucralose

Highly Processed Foods

Diet and Low-Fat Products: Crackers, Cereals, etc

Consuming unhealthy sugary products can actually cause you to be hungrier after consuming them, as they only temporarily satisfy. On your mission to lose weight, you have to be determined and take decisive measures.

It is important that you prepare your own food during your weight loss week as it limits your consumption of artificial sweeteners and junk food.

To reduce your sugar intake, you should drink more water, instead of drinking sodas. Even before snacking, you can drink water. In that way, you will commit to consuming your required serving of your snack instead of eating more than is needed.

Skipping meals is not advisable. When you skip meals, you deprive your body of the much needed nutrients and side effects can include, headaches, fatigue and low mental performance. In the long run, avoiding meals, increases the risk of acquiring health problems.

Take the time to have a proper meal. You have to make time and take a break from your work. Eating a meal while working or while distracted may cause you to eat less. Later, when you become hungry as you did not consume a proper meal, you may have the urge to eat food, not on your weight loss diet plan. Monitoring calories and carbohydrates is the last thing anyone is mindful of when quickly trying to satiate one's hunger. Therefore, you should have an allotted time for your meals.

You do not need to starve or skip your meals. The recipes in this book are easy to prepare, healthy and delectable.

Whether you prefer preparing easy meals or adventurous cuisine or eating exotic or traditional meals, there are a wide array of recipes for your selection. Also, if you are entertaining guests at your home, you can still adhere to your diet while preparing delicious meals for them. So savor every bite of your prescribed meal during your weight loss journey. Let us now look at the recipes.

Low Carb Breakfast Recipes

Strawberry-Banana Smoothie

(12 grams of carbohydrates and 54 calories per serving)

Servings: 8
Serving size: ½ cup

Ingredients

  1 peeled and sliced kiwi fruit
  1 cup of ice cubes
  1 (6 ounce) carton of vanilla low-fat yoghurt
  1 sliced medium banana
  4 cups of sliced fresh strawberries

Directions

Put into a blender banana, yoghurt, and strawberries and blend until smooth. As the blender is still on, put in one ice cube at a time, through the hole in the lid. Blend until the mix is smooth then transfer the mixture into 8 small glasses, top with some kiwifruit and serve immediately.

Cream Cheese Pancakes

(2.5 grams of carbohydrates and 344 calories per serving)

Makes: 4 pancakes

Ingredients

- ½ teaspoon of cinnamon
- 1 packet of Stevia
- 2 eggs
- 2 oz. of cream cheeses

Directions

In a blender, smoothly blend all the ingredients. Set aside for 2 minutes so that the bubbles can clear up. Grease a pan with butter or cooking spray. Transfer 1/4 of the batter into the pan. Cook for approximately 2 minutes until golden and flip and cook the other side for 1 minute. Do the same thing, with the rest of the batter. Serve with syrup and fresh berries.

Breakfast Burrito

(14 grams of carbohydrates and 179 calories per serving)

Servings: 4

Ingredients

 4 teaspoons of snipped fresh mint
 ¼ cup of dairy sour cream
 ½ cup of shredded Monterey Jack cheese (2 ounces)
 1 medium tomato, thinly sliced
 Nonstick cooking spray or cooking oil
 1/8 teaspoon of salt
 ¼ teaspoon of black pepper
 2 tablespoons of milk
 4 eggs
 1/3 cup of bottled chunky salsa
 1 cup of canned black beans rinsed and drained
 Bottled chunky salsa (optional)

Directions

Slightly mash the beans in a saucepan then add in 1/3 cup of salsa and heat over low heat. Cover and keep warm as you make the egg tortillas.

Whisk the eggs in a bowl then add in pepper, salt, and milk, coat a nonstick omelet pan with cooking oil or cooking spray. Preheat the pan until a drop of water sizzles, over medium heat.

Pour around a ¼ cup the egg mix into the heated pan then lift and tilt it to spread the egg mixture evenly on the pan. Return the pan to heat and cook for about 1 ½ to 2 minutes until the egg mixture is browned lightly on the bottom; do not turn the egg mix.

Loosen the sides of the egg mix using a spatula; then slide carefully onto a plate the browned side down. On one half of the egg tortilla, spread ¼ of the bean salsa mix. Top using some cheese and onion then fold into half then into quarters to form burritos. Garnish with remaining cheese and sour cream then drizzle with mint. If you would like, you can serve with some more salsa.

Low Carb Waffles

(3 grams of carbohydrates and 121 calories per serving)

Makes 1 full waffle

Ingredients

> ½ teaspoon baking powder
> 2 tablespoons of unsweetened almond milk
> 2 tablespoons of coconut flour
> 2 egg whites plus 1 whole egg
> Sweetener to taste, optional

Directions

Using an eggbeater or hand mixer, beat two of the egg whites to stiff peaks then stir in baking powder, coconut flour, unsweetened almond milk, 1 whole egg and sweetener. Heat the waffle iron to high heat then spray or grease it using nonstick spray. Pour the batter into the waffle iron and cook for around 3-4 minutes until browned. Serve and enjoy.

Herb-Bran Muffins

(22 grams of carbohydrates and 162 calories per serving)

Makes 10 to 12 muffins

Ingredients

¼ cup of cooking oil
1 cup of buttermilk
2 beaten egg whites
2 teaspoons of snipped fresh rosemary
¼ teaspoon of baking soda
½ teaspoon of baking powder
1 tablespoon of sugar
2 tablespoons of grated Parmesan cheese
1 cup of bran cereal
1 ½ cups of all-purpose flour
Non-stick cooking spray

Directions

Coat muffin cups with nonstick cooking spray lightly then put aside. In a bowl, combine cereal, flour, Parmesan cheese, desired herb, sugar, baking soda, and baking powder. Combine well then create a space at the center of flour mixture.

Mix together cooking oil, egg white and buttermilk in a bowl then pour the milk mix into the flour mixture. Stir until the mixture is lumpy and moistened. Scoop the batter into the muffin cups and bake for about 20 minutes in a 400-degree oven until golden. Leave the muffins to cool for around 5 minutes on a wire rack. Remove the muffins from the muffin cups and serve warm.

Shrimp-Artichoke Frittata

(6 grams of carbohydrates and 126 calories per serving)

Servings: 4

Ingredients

 3 tablespoons of finely shredded Parmesan cheese
 Nonstick cooking spray
 1/8 teaspoon of pepper
 1/8 teaspoon of garlic powder
 ¼ cup of thinly sliced green onions
 ¼ cup of fat-free milk
 2 cups of refrigerated egg product, thawed
 ½ (9 ounce) package of frozen artichoke hearts
 4 ounces of frozen shrimp in shells
 Italian parsley
 Cherry tomatoes, quartered

Directions

Defrost the shrimp if frozen then peel and devein it. Rinse the shrimp and pat it dry using paper towels, then halve the shrimp lengthwise. Set aside as you cook the artichoke hearts.

Drain and slice the artichoke hearts into quarters and put them aside. Mix together milk, pepper, egg product, green onions, and garlic powder and put aside. Coat lightly a large skillet with cooking spray and heat it until a drop of water sizzles. Put in the shrimp and cook for about 1-3 minutes until the shrimp becomes opaque.

Transfer the egg mixture into the skillet (do not stir), and put the skillet over medium to low heat. Once the egg begins to set, run a spoon or spatula round the side of the skillet, lifting the edges to let the egg liquid to run underneath. Continue to cook and lift the edges until the mix is almost set; the top side will be wet.

Remove the large skillet from the heat, and sprinkle some artichoke pieces equally over the top. Drizzle with some parmesan cheese and leave it to stand for about 3-4 minutes while covered until the top part of the frittata is set. Loosen the sides of the frittata and place it on a serving plate. Slice into wedges and serve then garnish with parsley and cherry tomatoes.

Baked Corned Beef Omelet

(5 grams of carbohydrates and 100 calories per serving)

Servings: 4

Ingredients

- ½ teaspoon seasoned salt
- 1 cup of heavy cream
- 1 (3-ounce) package of thinly sliced corned beef
- 1 tablespoon of green onion – chopped
- 1 cup of grated mozzarella cheese
- 8 large eggs

Directions

Preheat the oven to about 325 degrees then beat the seasoned salt, eggs and cream. Slice the corned beef into small pieces then add to the egg mix. Put in onion and cheese then pour the mixture into a greased baking dish. Bake while uncovered for about 45 minutes until the top is golden brown and set.

Bacon, Egg, and Kale Breakfast Salad

(14 grams of carbohydrates and 258 calories per serving)

Serving: 1

Ingredients

- 1 bacon slice, cooked and crumbled
- 1/8 teaspoon freshly grounded pepper
- 1 large egg
- 2 cups chopped Lacinato kale
- 1/2 cup halved grape tomatoes
- 1 1/2 teaspoons extra-virgin olive oil
- 1 1/2 teaspoons cider vinegar
- 1/8 teaspoon kosher salt

Directions

Pour water in a small saucepan and boil. Place a cold egg in it, reduce heat and cook for 6 minutes. Drain water, rinse egg with cold water, then peel it. In a bowl, mix tomatoes and kale, trickle vinegar and oil and season with salt. Toss mixture and then cover with bacon. Slice egg in half and place halves on salad. Season with pepper.

Greek Omelet

(6 grams of carbohydrates and 204 calories per serving)

Serving: 1

Ingredients

2 eggs + 1 egg white, beaten
1/2 teaspoon extra virgin olive oil
3 tablespoons red onion, diced
1/2 Roma tomato, diced
1 cup baby spinach
1 tablespoon reduced fat Feta cheese crumbles
1 tablespoon basil, chopped
pinch salt, to taste
pinch black pepper, to taste

Directions

With a 6-inch or similar size skillet, heat over medium-low temperature. Pour the oil in it, then add onion, spinach and tomato. Let it cook until spinach wilts and onions are tender. This should take about 2 minutes. Transfer the cooked vegetables to a plate.

With non-stick cooking spray, coat the skillet and add the beaten eggs. Flavor with black pepper and salt. Let the egg set for approximately 30 seconds. With a rubber spatula, loosen the egg's edges and slant the skillet up, marginally. Draw the eggs up towards the center of the skillet so that the uncooked part of the egg can run down in the skillet. Continue for about 2-3 minutes so that almost all of the uncooked part is cooked.

Add the cooked vegetables, basil and Feta cheese to one side when the egg is marginally uncooked. Fold the other side over to contain the filling. Cook for an extra minute so that the Feta cheese melts and inside cooks properly.

Quiche

(3 grams of carbohydrates and 111 calories per serving)

Servings: 6

Ingredients

- 1 cup low fat cottage cheese
- 2 cups liquid egg whites
- 1/2 cup broccoli, cooked and chopped
- 1/2 cup extra-lean ham, diced
- 1/4 teaspoon salt
- 1/2 cup Sargento Reduced Fat Sharp Cheddar Shredded Cheese
- 1/4 teaspoon black pepper

Directions

Heat oven to 375°F. In a sizeable mixing bowl, combine the ingredients. With non-stick cooking spray, coat a 9 ½-inch pie dish. Fill the dish with the ingredients and bake for about 45 minutes. When the middle of the dish is set, then it is completed.

Peppermint Patty Protein Shake

(7 grams of carbohydrates and 200 calories per serving)

Servings: 1

Ingredients

1/4 cup Designer Whey protein powder (vanilla or chocolate)
2-4 drops peppermint extract (or to taste)
1-3 packets Stevia (or 1/4-1 tablespoon sweetener of
choice)
1/2 cup fat free cottage cheese
2 tablespoons unsweetened cocoa powder
5-10 ice cubes (Depending on how thick you like it, use
less for a thinner consistency)
1/2- 1 cup water (Alter this according to desired consistency)

Directions

Put everything into a blender and blend until creamy consistency is attained.

Spinach and Mushroom Scrambled Eggs

(5 grams of carbohydrates and 137 calories per serving)

Servings: 1

Ingredients

- 1 cup raw spinach
- 4 mushrooms
- 21 g Laughing Cow light Swiss original cheese
- 1 egg
- 1 egg white

Directions

Dice mushrooms and add them and raw spinach to a non-stick pan over a high heat. Add one tablespoon of water to the pan and fry until mushrooms are cooked and spinach wilts. If needed, add more water until it evaporates. Remove and place aside.

In a small bowl, mix 1 egg and 1 egg white. Add 1 table-spoon of water and whisk. Cut a wedge of Laughing Cow light Swiss cheese into small chunks. Pour egg mix into the non-stick pan, using spatula to stir and scramble eggs. As it cooks, add the chunks of cheese. On a plate, arrange mushroom and spinach mixture and top with the mixture of scrambled eggs.

Ricotta, Tomato & Spinach Frittata

(7 grams of carbohydrates and 236 calories per serving)

Serves: 4

Ingredients

  small handful basil leaves
  100g ricotta
  6 eggs, beaten
  1 tablespoon olive oil
  1 large onion, finely sliced
  300g cherry tomatoes
  100g spinach leaves

Directions

Heat oven at 200C/180C fan/gas 6. In a sizeable non-stick frying pan heat oil. For 5-6 minutes cook onion until slightly golden and tender. Place the tomatoes in skillet and toss for 1 minute so that they become soft.

Take it off the heat. Insert basil and spinach leaves and toss so that they wilt a bit. Remove the contents and place in a greased rectangular baking tin approximately measuring 30 cm x 20 cm. Sprinkle ricotta over the vegetables.

Flavor the eggs with seasoning, whisk properly and pour onto the cheese and vegetables. Bake in oven for 20-25 minutes. When the mixture is set and slightly golden it is done.

Asparagus-Cheese Omelet

(4 grams of carbohydrates and 116 calories per serving)

Servings: 1

Ingredients

   1 tablespoon red sweet pepper slivers
   1 teaspoon snipped fresh parsley or basil
   non-stick cooking spray
   3 -5 thin spears asparagus
   3 egg whites, or 2 egg whites and 1 whole egg, or 1/2 cup refrigerated or frozen egg product, thawed
   1/8 teaspoon fresh pepper
   1 ounce desired flavor individually foil-wrapped spreadable cheese wedge that is cut up
   1/2 teaspoon olive oil

Directions

With the non-stick cooking spray, slightly spray a sizeable and unheated non-stick skillet. Insert asparagus and pan-roast over a medium-high temperature until browned and crisp. Occasionally turn. It should take about 7 minutes to cook.

In a medium-sized bowl, mix egg whites and pepper. Beat with a fork but do not let it become frothy. Over a medium-high temperature, heat oil in an 8-inch non-stick skillet, then add egg whites. Lower the heat to medium.

Use a heatproof spatula, and when eggs start setting, lift edges of egg white tenderly. Slant pan so that the liquid egg white can run under the set egg, and do so until egg is set and shiny. In the skillet, place the asparagus spears on half of the eggs. Cover with cheese in equal proportions. With the unfilled half of the eggs, fold over the cheese and asparagus. Skillfully slide the omelet out of the skillet and transfer to a plate. Use parsley and red sweet pepper slivers to garnish by sprinkling them on omelet.

Zucchini Tofu Scramble

(14.33 grams of carbohydrates and 130 calories per serving)

Servings: 6

Ingredients

  1/2 lb. extra firm tofu, cubed
  1 tablespoon vegetable oil
  salt & pepper
  1 large sweet onion, chopped
  6 cups zucchini
  2 -3 medium tomatoes, chopped

Directions

Sauté the onions in the oil until almost tender. Add zucchinis until just heated through. Add tomatoes and finally the tofu.

Yogurt-Filled Cantaloupe

(14.2 grams of carbohydrates and 101 calories per serving)

Ingredients

Servings: 1

1 cantaloupe
1/2 cup plain low-fat yogurt
10 blueberries

Directions

Cut cantaloupe in half and spoon out seeds. Save one half in fridge to use another time. Spoon yogurt into cantaloupe and add blueberries.

Prosciutto-Wrapped Melon

(8 grams of carbohydrates and 65 calories per serving)

Servings: 4

Serving Size: 3 pieces

Ingredients

> 1/4 ripe Galia melon (or cantaloupe or honeydew)
> 3 ounces chilled prosciutto

Directions

Cut melon in half, lengthwise and scoop the seeds out. Cut into four 1 ¼-inch wide wedges and remove the rind. Create two cuts the short way, across each wedge. You should have three pieces for each wedge.

Individually, cut every prosciutto slice in half, lengthwise. You should have two thin strips for every slice. Take a slice of prosciutto, and wrap it around a piece of melon. Do the same for the others. Put three pieces on a plate per serving. Serve cold.

Roasted Veggie Frittata

(8 grams of carbohydrates and 139 calories per serving)

Servings: 6

Ingredients

- 1 tablespoon olive oil
- 1/4 cup fresh parsley, chopped
- 1 teaspoon salt
- 4 eggs plus 6 egg whites
- 1/4 teaspoon cayenne pepper
- 1/3 cup finely shredded Parmesan
- non-stick cooking spray
- 3 medium red bell peppers, seeded and cut into quarters
- 4 garlic cloves, unpeeled
- 2 large zucchini, cut into 3-1/2-inch strips
- 1 medium onion, cut into 1/2-inch slices

Directions

Set the oven to 425° to preheat and position two oven racks in the center and lower oven placements. Select two shallow baking pans, line them with foil and spray cooking spray lightly on foil.

In one pan add garlic and bell peppers. In the other pan add the zucchini and onion. Use oil to brush vegetables. On lower rack, roast onion and zucchini and on center rack roast bell peppers and garlic. Roast them for 15 minutes. Take zucchini and onion from oven but reposition bell peppers and garlic to lower rack. Roast the bell peppers and garlic for an additional 10 minutes or until they char. Take them out of oven and set aside for 5 minutes.

Take the skin off of garlic and peppers. Thickly chop vegetables and garlic and put them in a sizeable bowl. Mix in ½ teaspoon salt and parsley. Lessen the temperature of oven to 350°. Select a 9 x 1 ½ inch circular cake pan and coat with cooking spray. In a medium bowl, whisk eggs, egg whites, cayenne pepper and the remainder of the salt. Mix egg blend into vegetable combination and stir shredded Parmesan in it. Transfer mixture to the cake pan and bake without covering for 45-50 minutes or until the center sets. Take pan out of the oven and let it cool for 5 minutes. Serve.

Smoked Salmon Breakfast Wraps

(14 grams of carbohydrates and 124 calories per serving)

Servings: 4

Ingredients

4   6 - 7 - inches whole wheat flour tortillas

3 ounces thinly sliced, smoked salmon (lox-style), cut into strips

1 small zucchini, trimmed

1/3 cup light cream cheese spread

1 tablespoon snipped fresh chives

1 teaspoon finely shredded lemon peel

1 tablespoon lemon juice

Directions

In a small mixing bowl, combine lemon peel, chives, cheese, and lemon juice. Paste the mixture properly and equally over tortillas. Leave a ½ inch border around the edges when spreading on the mixture.

Apportion salmon on the tortillas, positioning it on the bottom half of every tortilla.

Make zucchini ribbons by using a sharp vegetable peeler and draw it lengthways along, to cut very fine slices. Put zucchini ribbons on the top of the salmon. From the bottom of the tortillas, roll them upwards, then cut them in half.

Low Carb Main Meals

Stuffed chicken with Sherry Dijon sauce

(10 grams of carbohydrates and 347 calories per serving)

Servings: 4

Ingredients

- 4 (6 to 8-ounce) of boneless skinless chicken breast halves
- 2 teaspoons of fresh thyme (chopped)
- 1 cup of low-fat evaporated milk
- ¼ cup of dry sherry
- 2 tablespoons of grated Parmesan cheese
- ½ cup of low-sodium chicken broth
- 1 ½ teaspoons of cornstarch
- Fresh pepper and kosher salt
- 2 teaspoons of olive oil
- 1 clove of garlic, finely chopped
- ½ cup (2 ounces) of grated Gruyere cheese
- 1 teaspoon of Dijon mustard
- 2 cups (4 ounces) of fresh broccoli florets
- Cooking spray

Directions

Preheat broiler then coat a baking dish with cooking spray. Put some salted water in a pot and bring it to a boil. Add in broccoli and cook for about 5 minutes until the broccoli is crisp tender and bright green. Drain well and squeeze the broccoli well in paper towels. Slice the broccoli and place in a medium bowl with garlic and Gruyere.

Insert a knife into chicken breast and make a three-inch deep pocket then stuff each of the chicken breasts with even amounts of the broccoli mix. Coat the sides of the chicken breasts with thyme and oil, and season using some pepper and salt.

Over medium-high heat, heat a skillet for about 5 minutes until the skillet is extremely hot then put in the chicken. Cook the chicken until it becomes golden brown and cooked thorough, about 6 minutes each side. If the chicken begins to turn brown quickly before cooking fully, lower the heat to medium to cook thorough then transfer to a baking dish.

Meanwhile mix together stock and milk in a pot and season with pepper and salt then let it simmer over medium heat. Combine cornstarch and sherry together until smooth then pour into the sauce as you whisk frequently. Cook until the sauce becomes thick for around 2 minutes then remove from the heat and add in the parmesan cheese.

Top each of the chicken breasts with two tablespoons of sauce then place under the preheated broiler. Broil for 2-3 minutes until lightly browned. Leave the chicken breasts for some minutes then slice each of the breasts into half on an angle. Stir in the mustard into the remaining sauce and spread some of the sauce on each plate. Top the sauce with the halved chicken breasts.

Pistachio Crusted Salmon

(9 grams of carbohydrates and 295 calories per serving)

Servings: 4

Ingredients

- 4 (4-ounce) of salmon fillets
- 2 egg whites, beaten
- ¼ cup of buckwheat flour
- 6 tablespoons of hulled pistachios, finely chopped
- Cooking spray

Directions

Preheat the oven to about 400 degrees F then in a dish mix the flour and pistachios. In another dish, beat the egg whites then dip one side of the salmon fillets into the egg mix then press into the flour and pistachio mix. Repeat the same for the remaining salmon fillets then once done put the fillets nut side up on a baking sheet. Spray the top part with some cooking spray then bake for about 25 minutes.

Slow-Cooker Pork Tacos

(14 grams of carbohydrates and 399 calories per serving)

Servings: 8

Ingredients

1 cinnamon stick
2 bay leaves
Freshly ground pepper
4 pounds of (untrimmed), boneless pork shoulder cut into chunks
3 ¾ cups of low-sodium chicken broth
2 teaspoons of dried oregano, preferably Mexican
Kosher salt
1 tablespoon of cider vinegar
2 tablespoons of honey
3 tablespoons of extra-virgin olive oil
½ medium white onion, roughly chopped
2 to 3 chipotles in adobo sauce
4 cloves garlic, unpeeled
3 whole pasilla chiles
3 whole ancho chiles
Assorted taco toppings, for garnish
Corn tortillas, warmed, for serving

Directions

Place the pasilla chiles, garlic and ancho in a medium bowl then add in 2-3 tablespoons of water. Put the mix into a microwave and microwave for about 2-3 minutes until pliable and soft. Stem and seed the ancho chiles then peel the garlic and transfer them to a blender.

Put into the blender oregano, chipotles, onion, 1 tablespoon of salt, honey, 2 tablespoons of olive oil and vinegar. Blend until smooth then heat remaining tablespoon of oil in a skillet over high heat. Put in the chile sauce as you stir frequently for 8 minutes until fragrant and thick. Pour the broth in then reduce the heat and cook until slightly thickened.

Season the pork chops with pepper and salt then transfer to a slow cooker. Put in the cinnamon stick, bay leaves, and the sauce. Cover and cook for around 5 hours on high heat until the meat becomes tender. You can also cook the meat in a Dutch oven at 350 degrees for around 1 hour 45 minutes while covered. Get rid of the cinnamon stick and bay leaves then using a fork shred the pork and season with pepper and salt. Serve the shredded pork in the tortillas together with the toppings.

Lentil Soup

(55 grams of carbohydrates and 37 calories per serving)

Servings: 6

Ingredients

- ½ teaspoon of freshly ground grains of paradise
- ½ teaspoon of toasted cumin (freshly ground)
- ½ teaspoon of freshly ground coriander
- 2 quarts chicken or vegetable broth
- 1 cup peeled and chopped tomatoes
- 1 pound lentils, picked and rinsed
- 2 teaspoons of kosher salt
- ½ cup of finely chopped celery
- ½ cup of finely chopped carrot
- 1 cup of finely chopped onion
- 2 tablespoons of olive oil

Directions

Put olive oil in a 6 quart Dutch oven over medium heat then once hot put in salt, onion, carrot, and celery. Cook until the onions become translucent for around 6-7 minutes. Add in the grains of paradise, lentils, cumin, broth, tomatoes, and coriander. Stir to mix well then turn the heat to high and leave the mixture to boil.

Lower the heat to low then cover and cook for about 35-40 minutes until the lentils are tender. Transfer to a blender then blend until your desired consistency. Serve right away and enjoy.

Chicken and Mushroom Broth

(6 grams of carbohydrates 179 calories)

Servings 4

Ingredients

200g chicken, shredded

Bunch of spring onions, sliced with greens and whites separated

100g Portobello mushrooms, sliced

Juice and zest of 2 limes

2 teaspoons sugar

1 tablespoon Thai fish sauce

1 tablespoon Thai red curry paste

1 liter hot chicken stock

Directions

Pour the stock into a pot then add in fish sauce, curry paste, some zest and lime juice then stir. Bring this to a boil then add in whites of the spring onion and mushrooms then cover and simmer for around two minutes.

Now stir in the chicken and some spring onion greens then heat through gently and ladle into bowls then scatter with remaining lime zest. Serve this with extra sugar, fish sauce and lime juice.

Chicken broccoli salad with avocado pesto

(8 grams of carbohydrates and 320 calories)

Servings: 4

Ingredients

> 2 raw beetroots
> 100g bag watercress
> 1 red onion, thinly sliced
> 3 skinless chicken breasts
> 2 teaspoons rapeseed oil
> 250g thin-stemmed broccoli

Directions

Bring a large saucepan with water to a boil then add in broccoli and cook for around 2 minutes. Drain then stop the cooking process by pouring cold water. Heat a griddle pan then you can toss the broccoli in with the half a teaspoon of the oil ensuring you turn until charred then put aside. Now brush the chicken with oil then season and put into the griddle turning after a few minutes until it is cooked through then allow it to cool.

Now make the pesto. Pick leaves from basil and set aside around a handful to top the salad then you can put the rest into a food processor. Scoop the avocado flesh then add into the processor alongside walnuts, garlic, 1 tablespoon lemon juice, 2 tablespoons cold water and seasoning then process until smooth then transfer to a dish. Now pour the remaining lemon juice over sliced onion and leave it for around a few minutes.

Put the watercress onto a large platter then toss through with the onion and broccoli with lemon juice then top with beetroot and chicken and some basil.

Meat Loaf with Sour Cream-Mushroom Sauce

(10 grams of carbohydrates and 214 calories per serving)

Servings: 6

Ingredients

> 1/3 cup fat-free milk
> 2 egg whites
> 1 cup soft whole grain bread crumbs (1 1/3 slices bread)
> 1/4 cup chopped green onions
> 2 teaspoons dried Italian seasoning, crushed
> 1/4 teaspoon salt
> 1/8 teaspoon pepper
> 1 pound lean ground beef
> non-stick cooking spray
> 1 tablespoon butter
> 1 and a half cups sliced fresh mushrooms
> 1 clove garlic, minced
> 1/4 cup thinly sliced green onions
> 1 8 - ounce carton light sour cream
> 2 tablespoons all-purpose flour
> 3/4 cup cold water
> 2 teaspoons instant beef bouillon granules
> sliced green onions (optional)
> Pepper (optional)

Directions

Turn on oven to 350°F. Select a 2-quart rectangular baking dish and cover the inside with foil.

Choose a large mixing bowl and add egg whites and milk. Use fork to properly beat the mixture. Add 1/4 cup chopped green onions, breadcrumbs, Italian seasoning, 1/8 teaspoon of pepper and salt. Stir in the ground beef and blend properly. Mold the beef combination into a 7 x 4 inch rectangle in the baking dish and bake for 1 hour or until internal temperature is 160°F. Spoon fat off and leave meat loaf for 10 minutes. Afterwards, cautiously transfer loaf to a serving platter with the use of two spatulas. Drain fat off.

Spray a medium-sized skillet with cooking spray. Melt butter over medium heat in skillet, then stir in garlic and mushrooms to prepare the sauce. Cook until mushrooms are almost soft. This usually takes 4 minutes. Add ¼ cup sliced green onions and cook for an additional minute.

Stir in a small mixing bowl, sour cream and flour.

To the mushroom mixture, add cold water and beef bouillon granules. Mix sour cream combination into mushroom combination in skillet and cook. Stir until it is thick then cook and stir for an extra 1 minute. If required, mix in more water to thin. Dish up the sauce over meat loaf. Drizzle peppers and sliced green onions on it, if you like.

Grilled Cheesy Portabello Caps with Turkey & Sage

(8 grams of carbohydrates and 260 calories)

Servings: 4

Ingredients

- 1/2 teaspoon salt
- 1/2 teaspoon fresh Pepper
- 1/8 teaspoon ground nutmeg
- 12 ounces lean ground turkey
- 4 large portabello mushroom caps
- 1 teaspoon extra-virgin olive oil
- 3 oz Cabot White Oak Cheddar
- 1 shallot, minced
- 2 tablespoons fine dry breadcrumbs
- 4 teaspoons minced fresh sage leaves

Directions

Turn grill on and set to medium. Get rid of stems from mushroom caps, scrape out gills with a spoon and dispose. Lightly glaze with oil.

In a medium-sized mixing bowl, combine nutmeg, pepper, salt, sage, breadcrumbs and shallots. Combine turkey and knead so that seasonings are spread consistently. Divide turkey combination amid mushroom caps.

Put turkey-side-up on grill. Cover with foil or close lid. Grill until it is properly cooked; this should last 10-12 minutes. Put cheddar on it and cook until cheese melts for approximately 2 more minutes.

Baked Chicken with Artichoke Topping

(9 grams of carbohydrates and 215 calories)

Servings: 4

Ingredients

1 (15 oz.) can artichoke hearts, drained and chopped
1/3 cup reduced-sodium, fat-free chicken broth
3 tablespoons grated parmesan cheese
cooking spray
2 tablespoons fresh lemon juice
4 (4 oz.) boneless, skinless chicken breasts
1/2 teaspoon garlic powder
1/4 teaspoon pepper
1 tablespoon olive oil
1 clove garlic, minced

Directions

At 350 °F, preheat oven. With cooking spray, spray baking sheet. Insert chicken breasts flanked by plastic wrap or insert in a plastic freezer bag and pound the chicken breasts until ½ inch thick. You can pound breasts with rolling pin, mallet or any appropriate equipment.

Over the breasts, squeeze lemon juice, then flavor with black pepper and garlic powder and bake for about 25 minutes.

In the meantime, over a medium-high temperature, heat the olive oil in a skillet. Combine the garlic, cook for 1 minute then add the artichoke hearts and cook for 3 minutes. Pour in the chicken broth and for about 5 minutes let it simmer. Add the parmesan cheese.

Take chicken breasts from oven and place the artichoke combination over the chicken. Continue baking until chicken is prepared. This usually takes an additional 10 minutes.

Onion-Stuffed Pork Tenderloin with Chutney-Mustard Sauce

(11 grams of carbohydrates and 176 calories per serving)

Servings: 8

Ingredients

    1 tablespoon olive oil
    1/2 cup mango chutney
    2 teaspoons Dijon-style mustard
    2 1 - 1 1/4 - pounds pork tenderloins
    1/3 cup finely chopped sweet onion, such as Vidalia or Maui
    1/4 cup chopped golden raisins
    1 tablespoon snipped fresh thyme and/or Italian (flat-leaf) parsley
    1/2 teaspoon kosher salt
    1/2 teaspoon fresh pepper

Directions

On tenderloins, trim fat and cut lengthways down the center, almost reaching the opposite side. Do not cut through for it should be able to spread open.

In a mixing bowl that is small, add thyme, raisins and onion. Place this stuffing over tenderloins and fold each piece of meat together again. To fasten securely, use a 100% cotton, kitchen string and tie at 1 ½ - 2 inch intervals. Glaze tenderloins with oil.

If you are using a charcoal grill, lay out the hot coals around a drip pan. Check for medium heat above pan, place meat on grill rack above the pan. Cover and for approximately 25-30 minutes grill meat or you can insert an instant-read thermometer in the meat until it reads 145 °F - 155°F.

If you are using a gas grill, preheat it and lessen temperature to medium; adjust accordingly for indirect cooking. Grill per the directions as charcoal grill, with the exception that on a rack in a roasting pan, you will put the meat; position pan on grill rack over burner that is off. Remove tenderloin and cover with foil. Set aside for 5 minutes before cutting it.

In a small mixing bowl, blend mustard and chutney to be used as a sauce. Discard the cotton strings from meat. Slice meat diagonally with a sharp knife and add sauce to servings.

Blue Cheese-Topped Pork Chops

(2 grams of carbohydrates and 194 calories per serving)

Servings: 4

Ingredients

- 1 roma tomato, cut into 8 slices
- 1/4 cup crumbled reduced-fat blue cheese (1 ounce)
- 1 tablespoon snipped fresh rosemary
- 2 tablespoons bottled fat-free Italian salad dressing
- Dash cayenne pepper
- 4 5 - 6 ounces bone-in pork loin chops

Directions

Heat the broiler. Mix salad dressing and cayenne pepper in a small mixing bowl. Skim every side of the pork chops with salad dressing. On unheated rack of broiler pan, position pork chops. Make sure they are 3-4 inches away from the heat. Broil for 8-10 minutes or until they are finished (usually at a temperature of 150°F.) Midway through broiling, turn once. When ready to consume, on each pork chop, place two slices of tomato and sprinkle with rosemary and blue cheese.

Prosciutto-Wrapped Shrimp with Arugula Salad

(4 grams of carbohydrates and 248 calories per serving)

Servings: 4

Ingredients

8 cups lightly packed baby arugula (about 5 ounces)
16 raw jumbo shrimp (13-15 per pound)
8 very thin slices prosciutto (about 2 ounces), cut in half lengthwise to make 16 strips
2 tablespoons plus 4 teaspoons extra-virgin olive oil, divided
2 tablespoons lemon juice
1 medium clove garlic, minced
1/8 teaspoon salt
1/4 teaspoon freshly ground pepper, divided

Directions

In a large bowl, whip lemon juice, 1/8 teaspoon of pepper, salt, garlic and 2 tablespoons of oil. Place arugula into the mixture and toss. Peel and remove the main central vein from shrimp but leave the tails. Dry thoroughly, and use the rest of the 1/8 teaspoon of pepper to sprinkle on each side. Around each shrimp, wrap a piece of prosciutto.

Over a medium-high temperature in a non-stick sizeable skillet, heat 2 teaspoons of oil. Insert half the shrimp and cook. Turn once and cook for approximately 4 minutes. Lower the temperature to medium and do the same thing with the rest of the oil and shrimp. When done, serve the arugula mixture with shrimp.

Cottage Cheese Puff

(12 grams of carbohydrates and 205 calories per serving)

Servings: 6

Ingredients

    2 cups cottage cheese
    3/4 cup soft whole wheat bread crumbs (about 1 slice)
    1/2 cup all-purpose flour
    1/3 cup snipped parsley
    1/3 cup finely chopped green onions
    2 tablespoons margarine or butter
    1/4 teaspoon salt
    4 eggs
    1 tablespoon snipped parsley

Directions

Blend flour, 1/3 cup parsley, green onion, margarine or butter, salt, cottage cheese and bread crumbs in a medium-sized bowl. Select a larger mixing bowl and using an electric mixer set to high speed, beat the eggs for 5 minutes until thick. Slowly add the cottage cheese blend over the eggs, combining the ingredients by folding.

Place the egg blend into a 5 or 6 cup soufflé dish or casserole that is not greased. Set oven at 350 ° F and bake for 1 hour. To examine its completeness, place a knife close to the center and remove. If the knife emerges clean then, it is properly baked. Garnish by sprinkling 1 tablespoon of parsley.

Salmon Burgers with Pickled Cucumber Slaw

(5 grams of carbohydrates and 126 calories per serving)

Servings: 6
Serving Size: 1 salmon burger with 1/6 pickled cucumbers

Ingredients

Salmon Burgers:
1 pound fresh raw salmon, skin removed
1 teaspoon toasted sesame oil
1 red bell pepper, diced
1 tablespoon minced garlic
1 tablespoon soy sauce
1 teaspoon curry powder
1/2 teaspoon turmeric
1 teaspoon ground ginger
juice of 1 lime (about 2 tablespoons)
Pickled Cucumber Slaw:
1/4 small medium carrot, thinly sliced
1/2 small English cucumber, thinly sliced
1/2 shallot or 1/4 small red onion, thinly sliced
3 tablespoons rice wine vinegar
1 teaspoon white sugar
2-3 mint leaves, chopped

Directions

Make the cucumber slaw first by mixing the cucumber, shallot or red onion, carrot, vinegar and sugar in a small mixing bowl. Finely slice vegetables with a mandoline slicer, using the thinnest setting. Place in the refrigerator until later. Keep the mint leaves for later use.

Over a medium-low temperature, heat a skillet inserting the oil, then garlic and red bell pepper. Cook them for 8-10 minutes until they are tender. Allow mixture to cool.

Pulse salmon in a food processor until the consistency is like ground salmon or chop it up in small pieces. Place it in a mixing bowl and add the vegetables, curry powder, soy sauce, lime juice, turmeric and ground ginger. Make 6 evenly-sized patties and place on a baking sheet lined with parchment paper. Refrigerate to get firm. Set the oven at 425°F and bake for 5-7 minutes.

Drain the liquid from pickled veggies and set aside for usage. Serve the mixed salad greens, and place the salmon burger on it. Sprinkle some of the liquid from the pickled vegetable. Place some of the pickled vegetables on every burger and garnish with chopped mint.

Slow Cooker Chicken and Pepperoni

(4 grams of carbohydrates and 307 calories per serving)

Servings: 4

Ingredients

> 1 cup reduced-sodium chicken broth
> 3 tablespoons tomato paste
> 2 pounds boneless, skinless chicken breasts
> 1 teaspoon Italian seasoning
> 1/2 teaspoon basil
> 1/4 teaspoon red pepper flakes
> 35 turkey pepperonis, sliced in half
> 1/2 cup sliced reduced-sodium black olives
> salt, to taste
> black pepper, to taste

Directions

Put the chicken on the bottom of the slow cooker, and season the tops with pepper and salt, to taste.

In a medium-sized mixing bowl, stir together the chicken broth, tomato paste, Italian seasoning, and red pepper flakes, then pour over the chicken in the slow cooker. Add the pepperoni and the olives to the slow cooker.

Place the lid on. Cook on a high temperature for 3 hours or a low temperature for 6 hours, until the chicken easily disintegrates. Use two forks or tongs and shred chicken in the cooker. Stir it up, so that it soaks up the rest of the liquid, for an extra half hour.

Lemon Garlic Tilapia

(1.8 grams of carbohydrates and 175.2 calories per serving)

Servings: 4

Ingredients

    4 tilapia fillets
    1 tablespoon olive oil
    1 tablespoon butter or margarine
    juice of 1 lemon
    1 teaspoon garlic salt
    1 teaspoon dried parsley flakes
    dash of salt
    cayenne pepper to taste

Directions

Preheat oven to 400.

Spray a baking dish with non-stick cooking spray.

Melt butter in microwave. Add olive oil, lemon juice, garlic powder, salt and parsley and sauté for a few minutes. Pour over tilapia fillets in baking pan. Sprinkle some cayenne pepper on top of fish.

Bake in preheated oven for about 13 minutes, and broil for an additional 2-3 minutes.

Cauliflower and Broccoli Soup

(15 grams of carbohydrates and 124 calories per serving)

Servings: 4
Servings Size: 1 1/4 cups

Ingredients

2½ cups unsweetened almond milk
1/4 cup shredded Parmesan cheese
1 head cauliflower
1 head broccoli
1 teaspoon extra virgin olive oil
1 tablespoon minced garlic
1 shallot, thinly sliced
black pepper to taste
1/4 teaspoon salt

Directions

Remove the tough center of the cauliflower and broccoli. After the centers are taken out, chop them up. Place them in a large pot of boiling water and cook for 8-10 minutes until soft. Drain.

Over a medium-low temperature, heat a skillet. Place the oil, shallot and garlic in the skillet and cook until the shallots are tender. This should take approximately 4-6 minutes. In a big stockpot with the use of an immersion blender or high-powered blender, mix the milk, cheese, shallot blend and cooked broccoli and cauliflower. Mix on a high setting until mixture is smoothly blended. Use pepper and salt to season.

Cheeseburger Soup

(16 grams of carbohydrates and 207 calories per serving)

Servings: 8

Ingredients

- 2 small carrots, shredded (about ½ cup)
- 3 stalks celery, diced (about ½ cup)
- 1/2 pound lean ground beef
- 2 tablespoons unsalted butter
- 1 small onion, diced
- 1 tablespoon minced garlic
- 3 tablespoons white whole wheat flour
- 2 cups low-sodium chicken broth
- 2 cups skim milk
- 2 Russet potatoes, peeled and medium dice
- 1½ cups reduced-fat mild cheddar shredded cheese
- 1 tablespoon Dijon mustard
- 1 tablespoon Worcestershire sauce
- 1/4 teaspoon salt
- 1/4 teaspoon black pepper
- 1 tomato, diced

Directions

Brown the beef, over a medium-high temperature in a small skillet. Remove excess fat, by draining. Melt butter in a large stock pot over medium temperature. Cook carrots, onions and celery for no more than 6 minutes. Include the garlic and cook for an extra minute. Blend in the flour and cook for an additional minute. Whisk the milk and chicken broth in and allow the soup to boil. Reduce heat and let soup simmer. Stir in the potatoes and simmer until they are soft. This should take 15 minutes. Add ground beef, tomatoes, black pepper, Worcestershire sauce, salt, cheese and mustard. Cook for 5 minutes more.

Fire-Roasted Tomato Soup

(8 grams of carbohydrates and 60 calories per serving)

Makes 4 (3/4-cup) servings or 3 cups

Ingredients

1 1/2 cup (14 1/2-ounce can) diced fire-roasted tomatoes
1 cup fat-free chicken or vegetable broth
1/2 cup 1% or fat-free milk
salt and pepper to taste
1 tablespoon chopped fresh chives or scallion
1 teaspoon olive oil
2 tablespoons minced shallot or onion
4 quarter-size slices peeled fresh ginger
1 tablespoon chopped garlic

Directions

Over medium temperature, heat oil in a 2-quart saucepan. Include ginger, onion and shallot and cook for 1 minute until soft. Mix in the garlic and tomatoes and simmer until the blend thickens. This should take 4 minutes. Mix in the milk and broth. Let it boil.

When it has boiled, place soup in a blender or food processor and smoothly blend or process. Put mixture back in saucepan. Serve and garnish with scallion or chives and season with pepper and salt.

Low Carb Snacks

Almond thins

(86 calories and 3 grams of carbohydrates per 8 crackers)

Makes about 48 crackers

Ingredients

  1/8 teaspoon of onion powder
  1/8 teaspoon of garlic powder
  3/8 teaspoon of salt
  1 egg white
  2 teaspoons of granular Splenda
  3 ounces of almond flour, ¾ cup

Directions

Combine all the ingredients in a bowl and ensure that the mixture is moist and holds together. Place the batter onto a greased sheet of aluminum foil around 15*18" then cover the batter using a piece of wax paper sprayed with nonstick cooking spray. Roll the dough out to around 1/8 thick, ensure that you get an even thickness then you can also peel up the wax paper, and make the dough to get a shape that is as close as possible to a rectangle around 9*9" square.

Once the dough is nice and even, peel off the wax paper and using a pizza cutter, slice the dough into about 1-inch squares. Place the foil on an oven rack and bake for around 10-15 minutes at 325 degrees until golden brown. Look after the crackers to ensure that they do not burn. Immediately the crackers at the outer edges are quite golden, remove them and continue baking until the rest becomes golden. Once ready, break the crackers apart from the score lines and leave them to cool. Transfer them to an airtight container for a few weeks before eating them.

Jalapeno poppers

(5 grams of carbohydrates and 45 calories per popper)

Makes 16 servings

Ingredients

  8 slices thin bacon, cut in half crosswise
  4 ounces cream cheese, softened
  8 fresh jalapeños

Directions

Slice the jalapenos into half and scrape out the membranes and seeds. Fill each of the halves with some cream cheese about four ounces for each. Wrap each of the jalapenos with ½ slice of raw bacon ensuring that you start with the end at the bottom of the jalapenos.

Stretch out the bacon to ensure that it goes all the way round the chile once then tuck the ends of the bacon underneath. Place the jalapenos on a baking sheet lined with a foil paper making sure that the cream cheese side is facing up. Bake for about 20-25 minutes at 375 degrees. If the bacon is not yet ready, you can broil for some more minutes until brown.

Sauted peppers and onions

(7 grams of carbohydrates and 58 calories per ¼ cup serving)

Makes about eight ¼ cup servings

Ingredients

Salt, pepper and other desired seasonings, to taste
1 large onion chopped or sliced
4 medium green peppers, chopped or sliced
2 tablespoons oil

Directions

Heat oil in a skillet over medium-high heat then fry the onion and peppers until they become slightly browned and tender. Season the onion mix with pepper and salt to add flavor then serve.

Roasted Baby Carrots

(10 grams of carbohydrates and 74 calories per serving)

Makes about 4 servings

Ingredients

¼ - ½ teaspoon of salt
1 tablespoon of oil
1 pound of baby carrots

Directions

Coat a baking pan using a nonstick foil then place the carrots in the pan and sprinkle some oil and salt.

Toss to fully coat the carrots and spread them on the bottom of the pan into a single layer. Roast for 12 minutes at 475 degrees, stir them around, and bake for 4 more minutes then stir again. Bake the carrots for another 4-7 minutes until they are nicely browned and tender. Sprinkle pepper and salt to suit your preference.

Cauli Tots (Baked)

(5 grams of carbohydrates and 38 calories per serving)

Makes about 30 tots

Ingredients

Salt, pepper, onion powder (to taste)
1/3 cup of grated Parmesan Cheese
1 (12- ounce) bag of frozen cauliflower

Directions

Cook cauliflower while covered in a microwave for about 6 minutes then pour out the water and let it cool. Place the cauliflower into a food processor and process well, and then as you make the cauliflower into its shape, squeeze out any excess water from the vegetable.

Roll the mixture into balls about 1.5 inches thick then drop the balls into Parmesan cheese. Make the balls into tots by flattening the tops then if the mixture is still moist and does not hold together, put into the tot some Parmesan cheese and roll formed tots into the Parmesan cheese again to coat fully.

Put the cauliflower tots on a cookie sheet that is greased then freeze the tots for about 30 minutes before you bake them to help the tots hold their shape.

After 30 minutes remove the tots from the freezer then pre-heat the oven to about 400 degrees F. Bake the tots for 10 minutes while rotating them constantly to ensure even browning.

Cheese roll-ups

(2 grams of carbohydrates and 159 calories per serving)

Serving: 1

Ingredients

Marinara or pizza sauce, optional
Garlic powder
2 ounces mozzarella cheese, shredded

Directions

Place a non-stick skillet over medium to high heat then spread the mozzarella cheese to ensure that the entire bottom of the skillet is completely covered.

Drizzle using garlic powder to add flavor then after the bottom of the cheese has become brown, slowly start prying the cheese using a spatula.

Start by pushing and rolling the cheese from one side using a spatula up to the other side then transfer to a plate. Repeat the same for the remaining mozzarella cheese.

You can serve and enjoy or dip the cheese roll ups in pizza or marinara sauce.

Pineapple and Cucumber Guacamole

(4 grams of carbohydrates and 24 calories per serving)

Servings: 5

Ingredients

   1 cucumber peeled, seeded, and diced (½ inch)
   1/2 red onion finely diced
   1/2 cup cilantro chopped, divided
   2 fresh serrano or jalapeño chiles minced, including seeds, or more to taste
   2 tablespoons freshly squeezed lime juice
   3/4 teaspoon fine salt or 1 1/2 teaspoons kosher salt
   2 avocados or 4 small, halved and pitted
   1/2 pineapple peeled, cored, and diced (½ inch)

Directions

In a sizeable bowl, combine the lime juice, chiles, onion, salt and cucumber. With a knife, make light cuts in parallel lines in the flesh of the avocado, in a cross-hatch design but not though the skin of the avocado, only the flesh. Scoop the flesh in the bowl stirring tenderly, ensuring not to mash the flesh. Add half of the cilantro and lastly the pineapple. Season to your preference with the additional salt, chile and lime juice. Place guacamole mixture on a wide dish and drizzle the rest of the cilantro on top. Cover with a plastic wrap and refrigerate for up to 2 hours. Allow it to be served at room temperature.

Greek Yogurt Dessert with Honey and Strawberries

(11.5 calories and 2.8 grams of carbohydrates)

Servings: 4

Ingredients

12 strawberries, washed and roughly chopped (or any other fresh fruit)
1 (8 ounce) plain Greek yogurt
honey

Directions

Put a few large spoonfuls of yogurt into 4 small glasses or ice cream bowls. Drizzle each with about 1 tablespoon of honey. Add strawberries on top.

Broccoli and Cheddar Quinoa Bites

(70 calories and 3 grams of carbohydrates)

Servings: 24

Ingredients

　　1 tablespoon grainy mustard
　　salt, pepper and cayenne to taste
　　2/3 cup quinoa, rinsed
　　1 cup water
　　2 cups broccoli, chopped
　　2 cups cheddar cheese, shredded
　　2 eggs, lightly beaten

Directions

Bring quinoa and water to a boil. Reduce the heat, simmer until tender and the water has been absorbed, about 15 minutes and let cool.

Mix everything, spoon into mini muffin pans and bake in a preheated 350F/180C oven until lightly golden brown on top, about 15-20 minutes.

Kale Chips

(16 grams of carbohydrates and 110 calories)

Servings: 4

Ingredients

   1 tablespoon extra-virgin olive oil
   1/4 teaspoon salt
   1 large bunch kale, tough stems removed, leaves torn into
   pieces (about 16 cups)

Directions:

Position racks in upper third and center of oven; preheat to 400°F.

If kale is wet, very thoroughly pat dry with a clean kitchen towel; transfer to a large bowl. Drizzle the kale with oil and sprinkle with salt. Using your hands, massage the oil and salt onto the kale leaves to evenly coat. Fill 2 large rimmed baking sheets with a layer of kale, making sure the leaves don't overlap. (If the kale won't all fit, make the chips in batches.)

Bake until most leaves are crisp, switching the pans back to front and top to bottom halfway through, 8 to 12 minutes total. If you are baking a batch on just one sheet, check after 8 minutes to prevent burning.

Zucchini Chips

(49 calories and 4 grams of carbohydrates per serving)

Servings: 4

Serving size: 20 (Total number of chips that can be made: 80)

Ingredients

- 1 tablespoon extra-virgin olive oil
- 1/4 teaspoon salt
- 1/8 teaspoon onion powder
- 1/8 teaspoon garlic powder
- 1 medium-sized zucchini

Directions

Warm the oven to 225° F. Place parchment paper on two baking sheets.

Finely slice the zucchini with a mandoline slicer and place the slices on paper towels in a single layer. Cover them with more paper towels. Place a baking sheet over them for about ten minutes to absorb moisture. Gently coat parchment paper with oil. In a single layer, place the zucchini chips on baking sheets. Slightly glaze the tops with oil. Season with onion powder, garlic powder and salt and bake for 1 – 1 ½ hours. Midway through baking rotate. The zucchini chips should be crisp when baking is completed. Allow them to cool for 5 minutes, then serve.

Spiced Pumpkin Seeds

(90 calories and 8.9 grams of carbohydrates)

Servings: 8

Ingredients

2 teaspoons Worcestershire sauce
2 cups raw whole pumpkin seeds
1 1/2 tablespoons margarine, melted
1/2 teaspoon salt
1/8 teaspoon garlic salt

Directions

Preheat oven to 275° F (135° C).

Mix pumpkin seeds, margarine, salt, garlic salt and Worcestershire sauce. Blend properly. Put mixture in a shallow dish that is appropriate for baking and bake for approximately 1 hour. Mix intermittently while it is baking. Serve.

Tomato Salad with Fried Capers

(7 grams of carbohydrates and 103 calories per serving)

Servings: 8

Ingredients

3 tablespoons capers, rinsed

2 1/2 pounds heirloom tomatoes, cut into 1-inch wedges

1 pint cherry tomatoes, mixed colors, halved

2 tablespoons red-wine vinegar

1 tablespoon Dijon mustard

3 tablespoons chopped fresh tarragon or dill

1/2 teaspoon freshly ground pepper, plus more to taste

1/4 teaspoon salt

5 tablespoons extra-virgin olive oil, divided

Directions

In a bowl, combine 1/2 teaspoon pepper and salt, vinegar, mustard, tarragon or dill and beat thoroughly. Add 4 tablespoons of oil and continue to mix until mixture is well incorporated. Dry the capers by patting them properly.

With the balance of the 1 tablespoon oil, heat it over a medium heat and add the thoroughly dried capers. Stir and cook for 3 minutes until lightly browned. Remove and place on a paper towel to drain.

Allot cherry tomatoes and tomato wedges on the plates. Dribble with vinaigrette and place the fried capers on top. Use the pepper to season.

Baba Ganoush

(86 calories and 7 grams of carbohydrates)

Servings: 4

Ingredients

> 1 medium or 3/4 of a large eggplant
> 1 large clove garlic, grated or finely minced
> 1 lemon, juiced
> 2 tablespoons Tahini
> sea salt
> Optional: 2 tablespoons fresh cilantro, parsley or basil, chopped
> olive oil (for roasting)

Directions

Turn on the oven to high broil. If the settings allow you to, you can turn it on to medium. Inside of the oven, place a rack at the top. Cut the eggplant into rounds that are 1/4 inch. Sprinkle with sea salt and drain excessive liquid with a colander. Allow the salt to saturate the eggplant for about ten minutes. Slightly rinse and dry in the middle of two towels.

Place on a baking sheet and trickle olive oil and a pinch of salt on them. For about 5-10 minutes let them roast. Rotate them once or twice until they are golden brown and soft. Take them out, then pile and wrap them in foil to hold the moisture. After 5 minutes, peel the tender skin of the eggplant and place the flesh in a food processor. Combine a pinch of salt, tahini, lemon juice and garlic until it is creamy. Lastly, add the herbs to the processor and mix well. Season according to your preference. Serve with vegetables.

Easy chocolate cake

(237 calories and 7 grams of carbohydrates per serving)

Makes 2 servings

Ingredients

1 egg

1 tablespoon of water

2 tablespoons of butter, melted

3 tablespoons plus 1 teaspoon of granulated Splenda

¼ teaspoon of baking powder

1 tablespoon of cocoa

¼ cup of almond flour, 1 ounce

Directions

In a measuring cup, mix together the granulated splenda, almond flour, baking powder and cocoa then add in egg, butter and water and combine well using a fork or spoon.

Scrape the butter evenly down using a rubber spatula then cover with a plastic wrap. Vent the plastic wrap by cutting a small hole at the center then microwave on high for about a minute until set and moist on top. Cool the cake slightly and serve warm with whipped cream. You can also let the cake to cool completely and frost as desired.

Mini Pumpkin Praline Bites

(93 calories and 2 grams of carbohydrates per candy)

Makes about 10 candies

The filling

> 3 tablespoons of sugar equivalent in a substitute
> ½ teaspoon of cinnamon
> 1/3 cup of chopped pecans
> 1/3 cup of pumpkin
> 1/3 cup of cream cheese, at room temperature
> *The coating*
> 2 tablespoons of sugar equivalent in a substitute
> 1 teaspoon of sugar free maple syrup
> 2 tablespoons of unsweetened cocoa
> 2 tablespoons of heavy white cream
> 4 tablespoons of salted butter

Directions

Mix all the filling ingredients in a bowl then form walnut sized balls from the mixture. If the mixture is very moist, refrigerate before making it into balls.

Place the balls on waxed paper in a refrigerator for about an hour.

To make the coating, melt the cream and butter in a microwave for about 30 seconds while stirring after 15 or 20 seconds. You do not want to fry the butter and cream but rather melt them.

Add into the cream and butter mixture, cocoa, sweetener and maple syrup. Remove the mini cakes from the refrigerator then roll them in the chocolate mixture and ensure that they are coated thoroughly.

Let them cool on a waxed paper until ready to serve then keep the remaining cakes in the refrigerator.

Velveeta Fudge

(128 calories and 3.2 grams of carbohydrates per piece)

Serving: 36

Ingredients

2 cups of chopped nuts
2 teaspoons of vanilla extract
½ cup of vanilla protein powder
½ cup of unsweetened cocoa
5 cups of confectionery sugar
8 ounces of cheese
1 cup (2 sticks) of softened butter

Directions

Melt butter and processed cheese together in a saucepan over medium heat as you stir constantly to avoid the mixture from sticking and burning at the bottom of the saucepan. Remove the saucepan from the heat then in a mixing bowl, gently mix cocoa and powdered sugar to avoid the particulate from making a mess.

Add in the cheese and butter mix then sugar and cocoa mix, mix well then put in the vanilla protein powder and nuts. Stir to mix well all the ingredients together then pour the fudge into a greased pan and put in the refrigerator. Cut into squares, serve, and enjoy.

Watermelon-Yogurt Ice

(74 calories and 16 grams of carbohydrates per serving)

Servings: 8, ½ cup each

Ingredients

1 tablespoon of lime juice
1 cup of low fat vanilla yoghurt
4 cups of diced seedless watermelon,
about 3 pounds with the rind
¼ cup of sugar
¼ cup of water

Directions

Mix sugar and water in a saucepan then cook as you stir frequently until the sugar is dissolved. Transfer the mixture to a measuring cup and leave it to slightly cool.

Put watermelon in a blender or food processor in two batches and blend until smooth. Place the pureed watermelon in a bowl then add in lime juice, cooled sugar syrup and yoghurt and mix until well combined. Pour the mix into another bowl through a fine mesh sieve whisking to release all the juices from the mixture. Throw away the pulp.

Transfer the extracted juices into an ice cream maker and freeze; you can also pour the watermelon mixture into a metal pan and freeze for about 6 hours or overnight until it becomes solid. Remove the ice cream from the freezer and slightly defrost it for around 5 minutes. Break the ice cream into small chunks and put in a blender in batches and blend until creamy and smooth. Serve the ice cream immediately or place in a storage container and put in a freezer for about 2 hours.

Magically moist almond cake

(256 calories and 6.5 grams of carbohydrates per serving)

Makes about 12 servings

Ingredients

  1 cup of water, optional
  ¼ teaspoon of salt
  ½ cup of coconut flour, sifted
  2 teaspoons of baking powder
  1 teaspoon of vanilla
  ½ cup of heavy cream
  1 ½ cups of almond flour
  4 eggs
  1 cup of liquid Splenda
  ¾ cup of butter, softened

Directions

Put all the ingredients in a large bowl then beat using an electric mixer until blended well and creamy. If the batter is very stiff, add in a cup of water and mix to thin the batter a little.

Spread the batter in a 9*13" pan greased with some butter then bake for 30-35 minutes at 350 degrees until the cake is firm to touch and golden. Leave it to cool completely before serving. It is advisable to store the cake in a refrigerator, as the almond flour will make the cake to quickly get moldy at room temperature.

Frozen Chocolate-Covered Bananas

(100 calories and 6 grams of carbohydrates per serving)

Servings: 12

Ingredients

> 1/4 cup shredded coconut
> 4 large ripe bananas, peeled and cut into thirds crosswise
> 3/4 cup semisweet or bittersweet chocolate chips, melted
> 12 popsicle sticks

Directions

Directions for melting chocolate

Set the microwave for 1 minute on medium and melt the chocolate. Swirl every 20 seconds and continue to microwave. Another option is in the top of a double boiler over water that is hot but not boiling, place chocolate. Swirl until it melts.

Directions for dessert

Insert parchment paper or wax paper on a baking sheet. Into the pieces of bananas place the wooden popsicle sticks, ensuring that they are well inserted. Use a rubber spatula and cover each piece of banana with the chocolate that is melted. If you need to melt the chocolate again, do so. Drizzle the chocolate covered bananas with the shredded coconut. Put the bananas on the baking sheet and freeze for approximately two hours.

Crisp Spice Cookies

(50 calories and 8 grams of carbohydrates per serving)

Servings: 66 cookies

Ingredients

- 1 1/3 cups all-purpose flour
- 1/2 teaspoon ground ginger
- 1/2 teaspoon apple pie spice
- 1/4 teaspoon ground cloves
- 1/4 teaspoon ground cardamom
- 1/8 teaspoon cayenne pepper
- 1/3 cup butter, softened
- 1/3 cup mild-flavor molasses
- 1/4 cup packed dark brown sugar

Directions

In a medium bowl stir together flour, ginger, apple pie spice, cloves, cardamom, and cayenne pepper; set flour mixture aside.

In a large mixing bowl beat butter with an electric mixer on medium speed for 30 seconds. Add molasses and brown sugar. Beat until combined, scraping sides of bowl occasionally. Beat in flour mixture until just combined. Divide dough in half. Cover and chill dough about 1 hour or until easy to handle.

On a lightly floured surface, roll half of the dough at a time until 1/16 inch thick. Using a floured 2-inch round scalloped cookie cutter, cut out dough. Place cutouts 1 inch apart on an ungreased cookie sheet.

Bake in a 375° F oven for 5 to 6 minutes or until edges are lightly browned. Transfer cookies to a wire rack; cool.

Creamy Lime Mousse

(112 calories and 4 grams of carbohydrates per serving)

Servings: 6

Serving Size: ½ cups

Ingredients

1/2 teaspoon finely shredded lime peel

2 tablespoons lime juice

1 4-serving-size package sugar-free lime-flavored gelatin

1 cup boiling water

1 8 - ounce carton light dairy sour cream

1 cup frozen light whipped dessert topping, thawed

1/2 cup frozen light whipped dessert topping, thawed (optional)

lime peel curls or lime slices (optional)

Directions

In a bowl that is large enough, mix the gelatin and boiling water. Stir until gelatin dissolves. In the mixture, stir the lime juice and lime peel. Cool for approximately 10-15 minutes but do not let it set. Whip the sour cream into the mixture and then the 1 cup of dessert topping, mixing lightly. Transfer the mixture into six 6-8 ounce stemmed glasses and cover. Place in the refrigerator and allow them to chill for 2 hours or as long as 24 hours. Ensure that it is set. If you wish, you can garnish with the lime peel curls, lime slices and 1/2 cup of dessert topping.

Walnut Fudge

(134 calories and 2.2 grams of carbohydrates per serving)

Serves 12

Ingredients

3 tablespoons dark cocoa powder

2 tablespoons granulated stevia, or sweetener of choice, to taste

1 teaspoon vanilla

120g / 4.2 oz. butter softened

120g / 4.2 oz. cream cheese softened

40g / 1.5 oz. walnut pieces

Directions

Mix the softened butter and the softened cream cheese until there are no lumps.

Add the cocoa, stevia and vanilla. Mix thoroughly. Add the walnuts and gently mix.

Place into a lined dish, or plate. Put in the fridge to set. Slice and serve.

Peanut Butter & Pretzel Truffles

(64 calories and 5 grams of carbohydrates per truffle)

Servings: 20 truffles

Ingredients

1/4 cup salted pretzels chopped fine
1/2 cup natural crunchy peanut butter
1/2 melted milk chocolate chips

Set the microwave for 1 minute on medium setting and melt the chocolate. Every 20 seconds, stir it and continue to microwave. Alternatively, in the top of a double boiler over water that is hot but not boiling, place chocolate. Swirl until it melts.

Directions

In a bowl, mix the chopped pretzels and peanut butter. Afterwards place in the freezer for approximately 15 minutes. Take one teaspoon of the mixture and roll it into a ball. Do the same for the remainder of the mixture until you have 20 balls.

On a baking sheet with either parchment paper or wax paper as a lining, put the balls on it. Place into the freezer for approximately one hour, until hardened. Afterwards, in the chocolate that is melted, roll the balls and place in the refrigerator. Leave refrigerated for approximately half an hour so that the chocolate can set.

Pumpkin Cheesecakes

(128 calories and 12 grams of carbohydrates per serving)

Servings: 16
Serving size: 1 cheesecake

Ingredients

- 1 tablespoon lemon juice
- 1 teaspoon vanilla
- 1/2 teaspoon cinnamon
- 1/4 teaspoon nutmeg
- 1/4 teaspoon allspice
- 1/2 cup pumpkin puree (100% puree)
- 2/3 cup sugar
- 2 eight-ounce packages of 1/3 less fat cream cheese, softened
- 16 reduced-fat vanilla wafers
- 2 eggs at room temperature

Directions

Heat the oven to 300°F. Line 16 muffin tins with paper liners. In every cupcake liner put 1 vanilla wafer. Use an electric mixer to smoothly cream the sugar and cream cheese. Insert one egg to the mixture beating properly, then add the other egg, thoroughly whisking the mixture. When this is done, add the other ingredients and beat properly.

Distribute the mixture to the liners, so that the tops are nearly filled. For 25-30 minutes bake them or until set, noting that the middles may slightly shake. After baking, let them remain in the muffin tins on a cooling rack for 15 minutes. Then take them out of the tins, cover and place them in the refrigerator until chilled.

Pecan-Cinnamon Wafers

(63 calories and 7 grams of carbohydrates per cookie)

Servings: 4 dozen cookies

Ingredients

   1 teaspoon vanilla extract

   1 1/4 cups whole-wheat pastry flour

   1 teaspoon baking powder

   1/4 teaspoon salt

   1 cup thinly chopped pecans

   1 1/2 teaspoons ground cinnamon

   1/2 cup unsalted butter

   3/4 cup granulated sugar, divided

   1/4 cup packed light brown sugar

   1 large egg

Directions

In a mixing bowl, with an electric mixer on medium-high, beat butter, 1/2 cup granulated sugar and brown sugar.

Include the vanilla extract and the egg. Whisk the mixture thoroughly. In a medium-sized bowl, add baking powder, salt and flour and include it to the butter combination. Put the speed settings on the electric mixer to low, and whip until the mixture is properly blended. Stir in the pecans.

Separate the dough equally in half and for each part, use your hands ensuring that they have flour on them, to shape the two halves into a 6-inch round log. Place the round logs in wax paper, wrapping them properly and put them in the freezer for about one hour until they are solid. Set the oven to 350°F.

Take the dough from the freezer, uncover. For no more than five minutes let it stand at room temperature.

On a shallow plate, blend the balance of the 1/4 cup granulated sugar and cinnamon. In this mixture, roll the logs and slice into 24 cookies. The thickness of each cookie should be ¼ inch. On baking sheets that are not greased, position the cookies approximately, 2 ½ inches away from each other. For 10 -12 minutes, bake each batch separately. They should be lightly browned when done. Place them on wire racks so they can cool off.

Mocha Ice Pops

(54 calories and 7 grams of carbohydrates per serving)

Servings: 10 (3-ounce) freezer pops

Ingredients

2 tablespoons unsweetened cocoa powder
2 1/2 cups hot brewed coffee
4-5 tablespoons sugar
1 cup half-and-half
1/4 teaspoon vanilla extract
pinch of salt
Equipment: ten 3-ounce (or similar-size) freezer-pop molds

Directions

Whisk coffee, sugar to taste and cocoa in a medium bowl until the sugar has dissolved. Whisk in half-and-half, vanilla and salt until combined.

Divide the mixture among freezer-pop molds. Insert the sticks and freeze until completely firm, about 6 hours. Dip the molds briefly in hot water before unmolding.

Coconut Mocha Frappe

(120 calories and 2 grams of carbohydrates per serving)

Servings: 2

Ingredients

1 drop of coconut extract
1 packet stevia (3.5oz)
2 cups unsweetened coconut milk
1 packet instant coffee (about 2 teaspoons)
½ tsp unsweetened cocoa powder

Directions

In a large cup, add all your ingredients together. Stir well. Place in a shallow freezer safe bowl. Every couple of hours scrape the mixture with a fork. Once frozen, leave on the counter until it softens up a pinch. Pop into the blender and process.

Tiramisu Cake

(199 calories and 14.9 grams of carbohydrates per serving)

Servings: 4

Ingredients

- 1 tablespoon oat flour (ground oats)
- 1 teaspoon baking powder
- 1/4 cup coconut milk
- 1/2 cup quinoa flakes
- 1/2 cup liquid egg whites
- 1/2 cup vanilla whey protein powder
- 1 teaspoon of Stevia or preferred sweetener
- double espresso made with hot water

Directions

Blend the first six ingredients and bake in a bread loaf tin at 160°C (320° F) for approximately 35 minutes or until, when you insert a knife, the knife comes out clean.

When it is cooled, slice it horizontally to form three layers. Cut the end edges off of each slice and place the slices inside a Tupperware. Make a double espresso with hot water and mix it with a teaspoon of any sweetener of your choice such as Stevia or toffee flavdrops. Pour over slices.

Cream Ingredients

- 1/4- cup coconut milk
- 1 tablespoon espresso
- 1/4 cup light mascarpone
- 1/4 cup vanilla casein protein powder
- cocoa powder for sprinkling

Directions

Blend the first four ingredients. Add some of the 'cream' to the first slice, cover with the second slice, add 'cream' to the second slice, cover with the third slice, add more 'cream' and sprinkle with cocoa powder.

Pineapple and Avocado Ice Pops

(104 calories and 16 grams of carbohydrates per serving)

Servings: 6
Serving Size: 1 Popsicle

Ingredients

    20-oz can pineapple chunks in 100% juice
    juice of 1 lime
    1 ripe avocado

Directions

Slice the avocado in half lengthwise, remove the pit, and scoop the flesh into the blender with the pineapple (and the canned juice), and lime juice.

Blend until smooth and pour into 6 popsicle molds.

Mini Chocolate Cheesecakes

(61 calories and 8 grams of carbohydrates per serving)

Servings: 1 dozen

Ingredients

> 1 tablespoon 100% fruit jam, such as raspberry or cherry
> 1/4 cup semisweet or bittersweet chocolate chips, melted
> 1/2 cup part-skim ricotta
> 12 chocolate wafer cookies

In order to melt the chocolate, set the microwave for 1 minute on medium setting and melt chocolate. Every 20 seconds, stir it and continue to microwave. Or in the top of a double boiler, over water that is hot but not boiling, place chocolate. Stir until it melts.

Directions

Combine melted chocolate and ricotta in a small bowl. Spoon a scant 1 tablespoon of the mixture on each chocolate wafer and top with 1/4 teaspoon jam.

**Thank you very much
and good luck!**

Made in the USA
Lexington, KY
26 June 2016